Living a good and Healthy life after 40

Steps for Successful Aging I provide a framework for healthy living that cover your changing needs for every decade

Richard C.H. Yates Sr.

TOC

Stocking a Healthy Pantry Dietary Needs

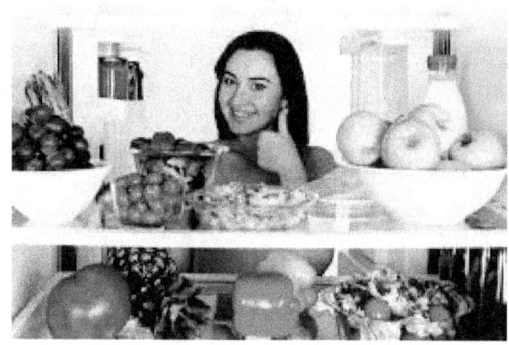

If you want to be healthy, it's important that you know what you are eating. Every day poses a challenge to eat healthy foods, because of tempting advertisements that you can see on TV, internet, and even on billboards.

The best way that you can prevent yourself from all these unhealthy eating, you have to discipline yourself by preparing your daily meals by yourself.

In this way, you'll know what goes in your body and this manner will also give you a sense of security in what you're eating.

Here are some suggestions for you to eat healthy by stocking your pantry with healthy food choices to satisfy your satiety and health.

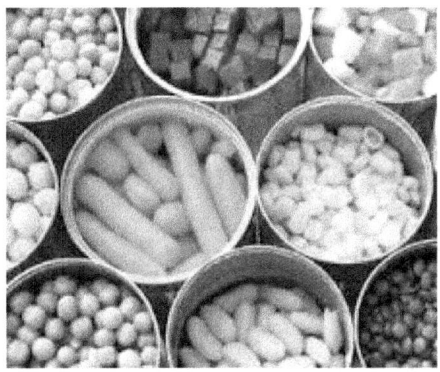

Healthy Canned Goods

Not all processed canned goods are bad for you. There are several canned products in the market that can be your healthy choices.

This includes canned tomatoes or tomato pastes, canned fat-free beans, canned soups for fiber, canned tuna and salmon, and many more.

These are processed foods, but the good thing about these products is that they tend to have more nutrient values canned with them.

Make sure that you read the labels of these canned products to see the calorie, sodium, and fat contents.

The lower fat content products are the healthier ones. Don't be afraid to stock up your pantry with these food choices that you can definitely enjoy.

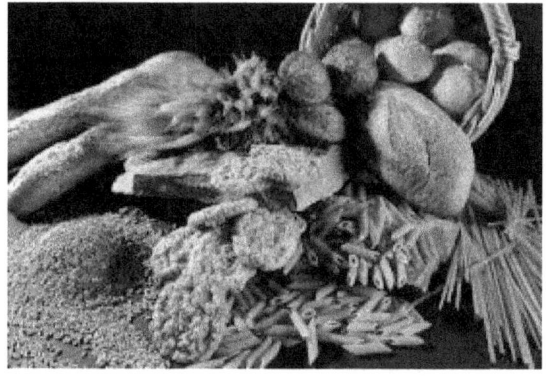

Healthy Grains

Whole wheat cereal is the most common healthy choice for whole grains today, because it's so easy and fast to prepare and eat during breakfast. Health-conscious people are also stocking their pantries with whole wheat pastas, whole wheat flour, rolled oats, brown rice, and yellow cornmeal. These are the healthy grains that will satisfy your appetite as well as your cravings without the guilt.

Whole wheat products are rich in fiber, nutrients, and are easily digested by the body. Stock up your pantry with these healthy grains and cook your favorite meals anytime of the day.

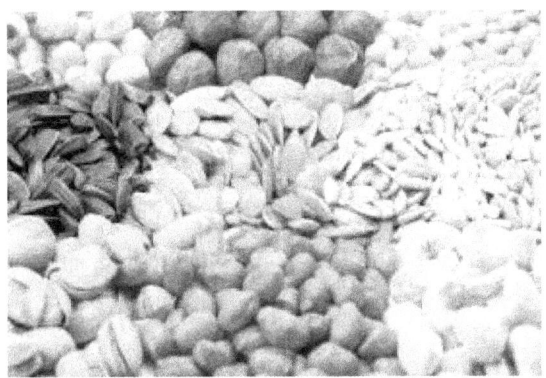

Nuts and Seeds

Some of the preferred nuts and seeds are walnuts, almonds, dry roasted peanuts, and sesame seeds.

These favorite nuts and seeds are used to add flavor to green salads and healthy cooked dishes.

You can give your own prepared meals a boost in taste with the nuts and seeds from your healthy pantry.

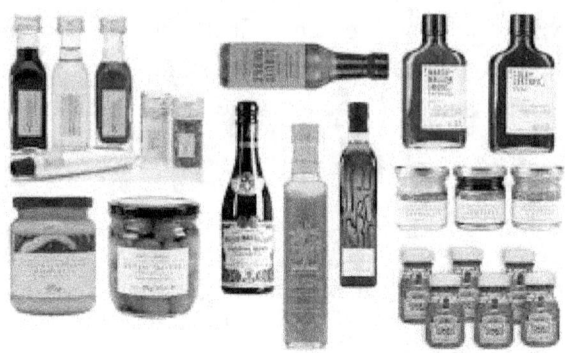

Healthy Oils and Condiments

Canola and olive oils are two of the healthiest choices of cooking oils. Make sure that you pantry includes these oils rather than using the regular oil that is sold in the market.

You can also use these oils as salad dressings or baking ingredients.

Asian condiments are also very healthy to use for cooking, such as vinegar, soy sauce, hoisin sauce, and oyster sauce.

You can also include barbecue sauce, mustards, and reduced-fat mayonnaise in your pantry for your salad dressings and meat sauces. These products don't only make your dishes delicious, but they also improve your health as you age.

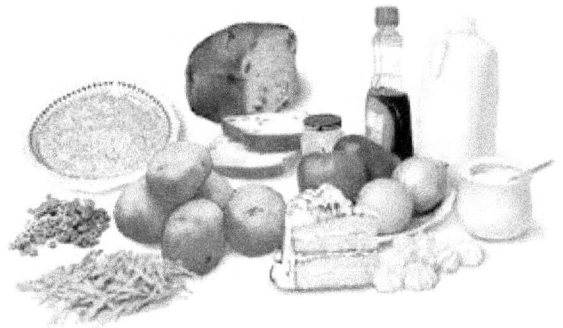

Refrigerator Stocks

Meat, fish, chicken, and other food products are important part of a healthy and balanced diet.

So make sure that you stuff your refrigerator with these products. These protein-rich foods will build your body in a way that you need every day.

Don't hesitate to prepare and eat these food stocks. Milk, cheeses, and butter should also be present in your refrigerator as they are good addition to certain main dishes and tasty snacks.

Fruits and vegetables are also very essential for your everyday diet plans, so ensure that you have enough of these food choices to satisfy your daily needs.

Having these food products ready in your pantry will save you time and effort from going to the supermarket again and again.

It's time for you to update and give your pantry a healthy makeover. Don't waste your time and money into stocking up unhealthy food choices that can be bad for your health.

If you want to be healthy and live long, you have to start your balanced diet plans today before you suffer the consequences.

It's easy, exciting, and more fun than you thought it would be to plan out your meals every day.

Be wise in buying products to stock your pantry. It is worth your whole life and your family's health depends on that wise buying, too.

You can have the best tasting food with the healthiest effect when you plan your healthy eating habits well. So, get those pantries ready for your next healthy food choices.

4 Exercises Every Person over Age 40 Should Do

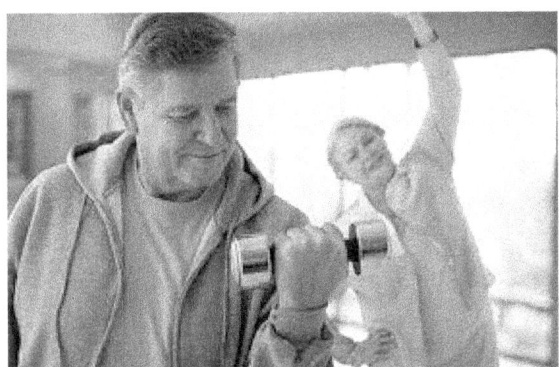

Just because you are getting older doesn't mean you can't life a long and healthy life. You can!

And it all starts with eating right and exercising on a regular basis. Staying fit has been proven to help you live a longer, fuller life. And that's what we all want right? Of course we do.

With this article I am going to share with you 4 types of exercises you should do if you are over the age of 40. They will all help you stay strong as you gracefully age.

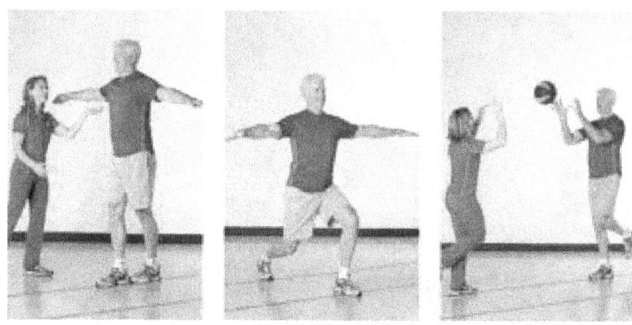

Balance Exercises

Many people start to lose their balance as they get older. As a matter of fact, over 2 million senior citizens fall every year.

Of those, close to 700,000 ends up in the hospital due to injury.

Falls are nothing to play with. A freak fall can lead to hip injuries, fractures and in more serious cases head injuries. But here's the good news!

You can reduce your chances of falling by working on your balance. Here are two simple balance exercises you can do right at home.

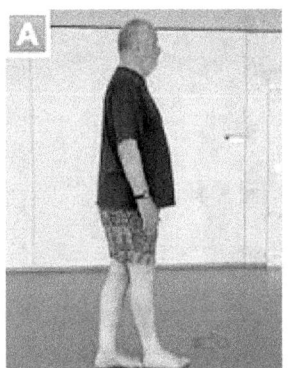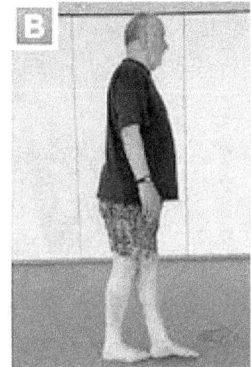

Walk Heel to Toe

This exercise is similar to walking on a tight rope. You will place one foot right in front of the other so that your heel and your toes are touching.

Put your arms out to your side and look straight ahead at a target. This can be anything.

With your eyes fixed on the target start walking. Take your time and walk heel to toe. Try to do at least 20 steps if you can't start with 10 and work your way up.

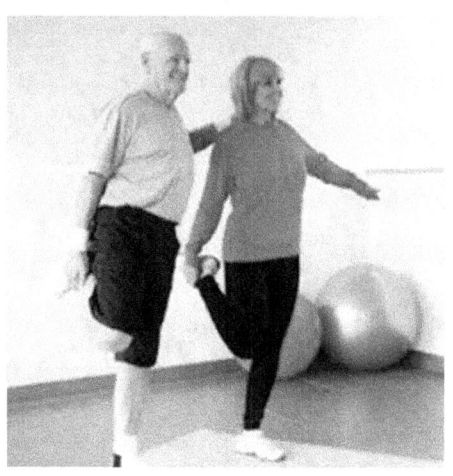

Stand On One Foot

Standing on one foot is a great way to improve your balance. Grab a chair, or something sturdy, you can use for balance. Place one hand on the chair and slightly lift up one leg. Hold it there for 10 seconds, relax and then do it again. Repeat this 10 to 15 times with each leg.

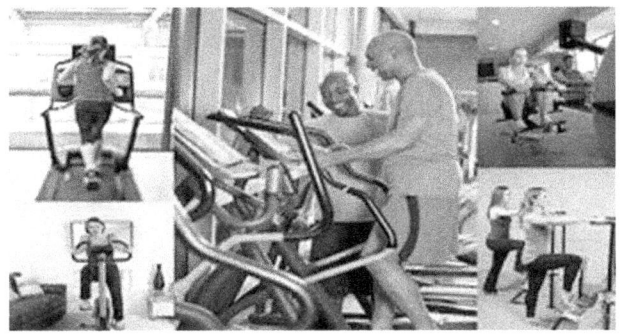

Endurance Exercises

Endurance exercises are very important as they help with circulation and breathing. As you get older you sometimes suffer from low energy levels.

Endurance exercises can help with that. Some great endurance exercises include swimming, walking, gardening and playing tennis. Start off slow and work your way up.

If you haven't worked out in a while start with 5 minutes. As you get stronger you can work your way up to 10 minutes and then ultimately 30 minutes. Doing this 3 to 4 times a week will have a dramatic impact on your overall health.

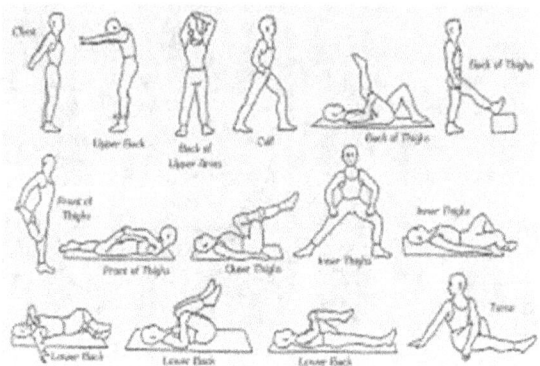

Strength Exercises

Once you reach the age of 50 you will start to lose up to 2% of your muscle mass every year.

When you lose muscle mass you also lose bone strength. This can lead to both balance and mobility problems. And that's why strength exercises are so important.

Especially if you want optimal health over the age of 40. Strength exercises involve lifting light weights. If you don't have any weights you can use items you already have in your home such as canned foods.

One strength exercise you can do is overhead arm raises. Take two cans of soup, or whatever you have, and sit down in a sturdy chair that does not have arms.

Make sure your feet are shoulder width apart and flat on the ground. Place the cans or weights if you have them, up to your shoulders. When you are ready to begin the exercise take a slow deep breath and push the weights up over your head.

Hold for one second and bring it back down. As you lower your arms breathe in. Do these as many times as you can? This exercise can also be done standing up.

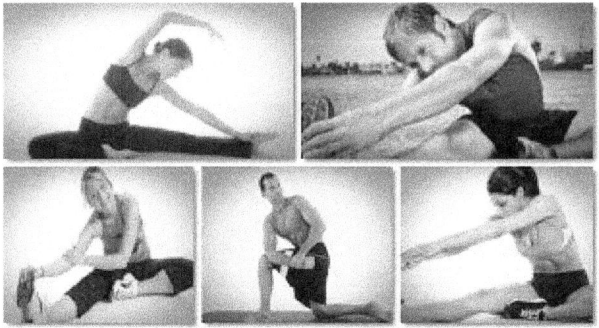

Flexibility Exercises

Last but not least we will talk about flexibility exercises. Sometimes as we get older it becomes harder for us to do simple things such as reach up to grab something.

Or an even better example is having a hard time looking over your shoulder as you are trying to back your car out of a parking spot. Does that sound familiar? Flexibility exercises will help with that.

Flexibility exercises are nothing more than stretching exercises. Stretching helps with your range of motion.

It also helps you stay limber. Yoga is a great flexibility workout. It works every part of your body and it builds strength and endurance in the process. You can do yoga at your local gym or you can buy a yoga DVD and do it from home.

How persons over 40 can stimulate new brain activity to help prevent the loss memory

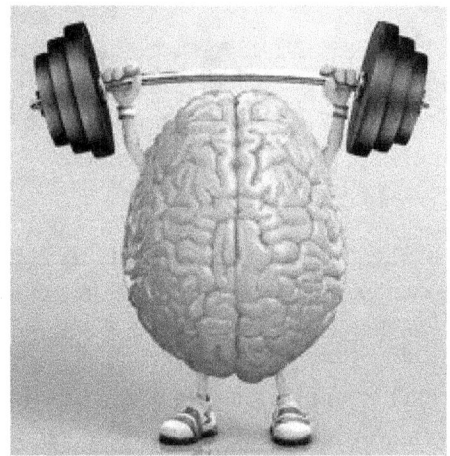

Life after 40 is burdensome to some people because, it is at this period that they start experiencing memory loss. There are many reasons that lead to the degradation of memory.

They include health problems, drug abuse, and depression, among others. The following is an instructive guide on how persons over 40 can stimulate new brain activity to prevent memory loss.

Travel has been found to stimulate the brain by introducing it to new experiences. It is worth mentioning that the human ancestors received tremendous brain stimulation through their nomadic lifestyle.

This is what resulted to the rapid evolvement of the human race.

Persons over 40 should, therefore, avoid sedentary lifestyles if they intend to avoid memory loss. Vacations to distant lands, hikes and trips should be taken regularly to engage the brain's memory center.

Depression is common in persons over 40 because they tend to live less social lives. Moving house, the loss of a loved one, retirement or a serious medical diagnosis are also major causes.

Depression has been found to mimic memory loss and make concentration difficult. It is important for persons over 40 to learn to adjust, stay close to persons who make them happy and in extreme cases attend counseling or therapy.

Getting organized immensely stimulates new brain cells and prevents memory loss. This is because it is easy for persons to be forgetful if their notes are not organized or where the homes are cluttered.

This makes it necessary to write down appointments, special events and tasks in a notebook. It is useful for such persons to read aloud each entry as it is written down because it helps cement it in their memory.

A to-do list item is invaluable because each completed task is marked so as to easily identify those that are pending. It is also important to set aside a specific place to keep keys, wallets, medication, prescription eyeglasses and other essential items.

Exercise has been found to lead to an improvement in cognitive function, in addition to, keeping the body fit and disease free. Persons over 40 are advised to engage in moderate exercises so as to heighten the speed at which their brains processes information, which also prevents memory loss. Playing golf has been associated with an improvement in sensorimotor control.

Musical training especially through instrumental musical activity and practice is helpful in the preservation of memory for persons over 40.

Musical training has been scientifically studied and found to increase the performance of memory cells in the brain as well as increasing a person's lifespan.

The brain's memory area should be considered as a muscle that needs exercise to keep fit. Persons over 40 are advised to stimulate it by playing scrabble, bingo, doing crossword puzzles or learning a new language.

These have found to be crucial because they trigger the brain's strategic thinking. Watching television should be minimized since it sends the brain to a neutral state.

Persons over 40 are advised to make sure that their vitamin B12 intake is sufficient. Due to the reduced nutrient absorption rates experienced by persons at such ages, supplementation through monthly injections may be necessary. Smokers and persons who take alcohol are particularly at risk because these tend to further reduce absorption rates.

The vitamin is useful in promoting healthy functioning of the brain and protecting neurons. Its absence in the body can lead to memory loss and irreversible brain damage.

Neurologic exercises have been found to be very helpful in the development of memory. It is necessary to include one of more of the body's common senses in everyday tasks.

These include washing hair or wearing clothes with the eyes closed or visual communication during meal times as opposed to verbal communication.

One can also use a combination of two senses such as smelling flowers while listening to music or taping fingers while listening to the rain. Daily routines should be broken in order by spontaneously trying out a new route to work or shopping at a new store.

Dehydration should be avoided completely since it can cause memory loss, confusion, drowsiness and symptoms that mimic dementia. Water intake should be included in one's diet. It is recommended that 6 to 8 glasses are taken on a daily basis.

Getting enough sleep results to memory consolidation. This is the process of the formation and storage of memories for future retrieval.

Sleep also aids neuron formation, which is important for sharpened memory, increased concentration and better decision making. Insufficient sleep can result to depression, which is associated with memory loss.

In conclusion, persons over 40 should stimulate brain activity to prevent memory loss because neurologists have found that memory loss is normal as a person ages.

It is referred to as associated memory impairment or age-related memory impairment, and can be considerably reduced by engaging the brain through mental and physical activity, avoiding depression and a healthy diet.

How Social Connections can help you

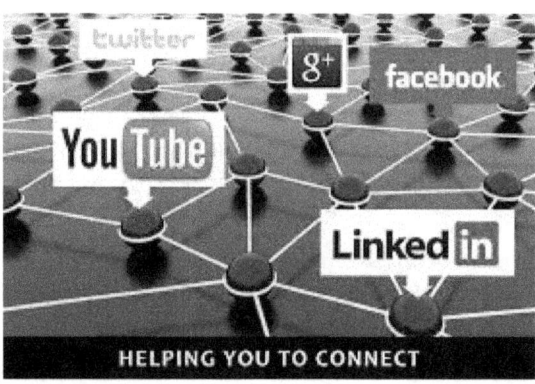

When you're getting advanced in years, it's easy to give up social connections and focus on yourself and your family.

However, recent studies show that strengthening your social connections with families, friends, and colleagues maintains a healthy outlook in life. You become more open to enjoy life and interact with people. It doesn't only maintain a healthy outlook in life, but it also affects your emotional and mental stability. Here are some useful tips on how to effectively strengthen your social connections to maintain your sense of daily purpose in life.

Take Good Care of Your Own Self

This is the crucial step that you need to take before you can even strengthen your social connections. Your physical health and your emotional, mental, and social health are interrelated. When your body is healthy and strong, you can do a lot more fun activities with your family and friends.

When you're doing interesting events along with social interactions with people, your body goes into a positive state and your organs, like heart, brain, and many others become more active, thus maintaining a healthy physical status than you'll ever know.

When you eat healthy, exercise regularly, and maintain a good personal hygiene, you also become more confident with yourself to socialize with people. That's why taking care of your own self is the first measure that you should not miss.

Communicate with your Family and Friends Often

Sometimes, people are too busy to talk to each other. However, the positive effects of these social interactions are a good contribution to your total health. Spend some time to call your family and friends from time to time.

Even a small talk on the phone can energize your social, mental, and emotional health. Don't take for granted all those little phone calls from a friend, because communicating with your close ties can build more confidence and security in you.

People who have known you for a long time occupy a big part in your being and talking to them ignites the love and trust that you've built with them. You will become more confident, reassured, and you will feel that good sense of belongingness again.

Practice the habit of visiting your mom's house or your friend's apartment and bring some food to share while having a good long conversation with them. As you grow old, it's rewarding to know that you have a family and friends that you can share your life with.

Plan Fun and Exciting Activities with your Family and Friends

Go on a date with your family or friends. Whether it's a movie date, a coffee date, or fun sports that you all enjoy, it's always worth it.

This will even teach you how to organize a small event with your close allies. You can also invite your friends over to your house. Prepare a home-cooked dinner and enjoy a karaoke night together.

The enjoyment that you get from all of these activities will enhance your positive outlook in life. Nothing is boring in life when you're getting old; it depends on how you approach it.

Make sure that you plan out fun and exciting activities regularly, like once a month or every other month. In this way, you are not only helping yourself, but you are also helping other people to stay young and positive as well.

Participate in Charities and Beneficial Events

One best way to feel the satisfaction of helping people is through your acts of kindness. When you actively participate in charities, in school volunteering jobs, and church projects, you also strengthen your social connections with people that can help you fulfill your sense of purpose in life.

You can explore more charitable institutions and organizations to help out with their beneficial works. You can even invite your family and friends to participate in these self-fulfilling events, too. Be thankful of your life and share this gratefulness to other people that are in need of your help.

Doing these useful tips will refresh your physical, emotional, mental health. There are more interesting activities that you can plan out and enjoy.

There's no limit in discovering more ways to interact with people and improve your healthy outlook in life. Seek more opportunities to talk and reach out to more people around you.

Online networking sites can also help you communicate with a lot more friends, both old and new. The best thing about having a positive outlook in life is you gain more friends in the process.

Medicate Wisely While Paying Attention to Aches and Pains

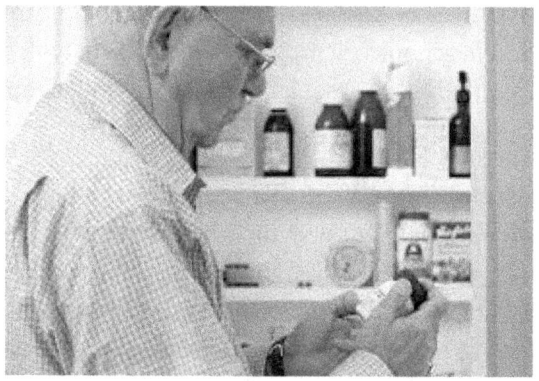

Pains and aches are common and usually caused by strains, sprains, illness, injury, fatigue or overuse of a body part. There are a wide range of medications prescribed for treatments of pains.

It is important to medicate wisely because some types of medications can have side effects and even prove life-threatening. There are some important things to know when it comes to using medications for relieving pains and aches.

Know the Type of Pain

You should first identify the type of pain. A simple pain will go away on its own even without any treatment or medication. For example, if you are not used to exercising then a long walk will cause pain in leg muscles.

If you do not lift weight regularly then lifting lots of weight on one day can cause pain in joints. If this type of pain is not severe then it will go away on its own.

If you started a new exercise regimen then continue with it and your pain will slowly go away in a few days. However, if you experience pain not caused by any such activity of if it is a severe pain that affects your general activity then you need medication.

Home Remedy, OTC Medicine or Doctor

If you are able to identify that it is a simple and temporary pain then simple home remedies like massage, hot water treatment, and taking rest may be sufficient to get complete relief.

If the pain is caused by an activity that you are not used to doing then you can try over-the-counter (OTC) pain relievers.

This type of pain must go away within a few days after taking such medicines. If it continues for a few days even after taking an OTC medicine then you need to consult a doctor. Ideally, you must take any medicine only after consulting a doctor.

Things to Remember When Choosing an OTC Pain Reliever

A medicine may be available in different strengths and formulations. You should never underestimate the potency of a medicine. First read complete information on its package before using it. Follow the instruction related to the dosage. Using a medicine of higher potency is not going to get you quicker relief. Take your dosages only at the recommended time intervals. If in doubt, start with the lowest dose amount recommended.

Avoid Long-Term Use of Any Pain Reliever

Use of any pain reliever must be temporary. Long-term uses of pain relieving medications for months and years can cause serious problems like liver damage. You should also avoid taking more than one pain relievers at a time.

Medicine interactions can cause serious problems. Some medicines react adversely with alcohol. If you are already on medication for an illness then take additional medication only after consulting your doctor.

Tackle the Root of the Problem

If you do not solve the main problem that is causing the pain then no medication is going to be effective.

The pain could be because of eyes and neck strain. Overuse of muscles can cause severe pain. Dehydration, fatigue, headache, tension and stress are also known to cause pain and body aches.

Sometimes, the pain could be because of an illness like cold. In such a case, you do not have to take any pain reliever; just treat the main illness and your body aches will go away as you are cured.

Time When You Need Prompt Medical Care

If you suddenly experience severe pain without any prior warning then you may need immediate medical care. A person, who is paralyzed, faces breathing difficulty or starts vomiting should be taken to the hospital immediately.

Treating Chronic Pain

A pain that does not go away with simple medication even after three months of treatment is classified as chronic pain. It can be continuous, intermittent or come in episodes.

It could be caused by an injury, accident or illness. It can happen even when the person has recovered from the health problem.

Any medication in such cases should be taken only after consulting a doctor. If this type of pain is caused by work-related causes then the person may even be advised to switch to another job.

Alternative pain relievers and natural pain remedies should be used only for simple pains. In case of a severe pain, the patient needs to consult a doctor immediately.

Some pains are a sign of serious disease that can be identified only after undergoing different types of checkups.

Healthy living every day: medicate wisely while paying attention to aches and pains. A regular exercise regimen and healthy lifestyle can help avoid most types of pains and aches to a great extent.

Take care of your skin

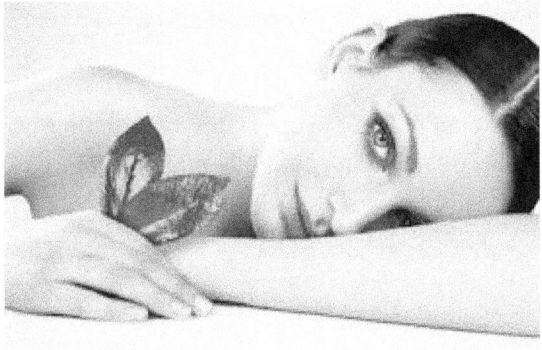

Everybody grows older, but on some people it is more evident than on others. There are lots of reasons for this discrepancy.

Among them are heredity, environment, habits and diet. It is important to realize that you have control over three out of four of these factors.

In this article, we will discuss some of the easily changeable bad habits that promote premature aging. Read on to learn how to take care of your skin to be healthy looks and most beautiful.

Sleep and excellent hydration are the top beauty products to prevent aging. Getting a full eight hours of good sleep every night will leave you rested and refreshed.

You will not have to worry about bags under your eyes, and your skin will have plenty of opportunity to recover from environmental challenges such as pollution and UV rays.

Staying hydrated will help your skin stay wrinkle free. It will also help every system in your body perform at optimum levels for overall beauty.

Be sure to remove your makeup and wash your face before bed every night. This is a lifelong beauty tip that will do more to keep your skin beautiful than almost any other topical treatment.

When you sleep with makeup and environmental contaminants on your skin they become ground in and cause all manner of irritation. A thorough washing and cleansing is best. If you are just too tired, clean your face with cotton balls and witch hazel and follow up with aloe Vera gel for light overnight moisture and nourishment.

 When you moisturize, exfoliate and apply masks to your face be sure to include your neck and throat and the backs of your hands.

If you take good care of your face but neglect these areas, the contrast will be very apparent. Nothing is more aging to your appearance than a wrinkly neck or hands that are riddled with liver spots.

Choose your beauty products carefully. Once you have settled on a particular product, be sure to give it a fair chance before changing your mind and switching to another product.

It takes your skin a little time to adjust, and part of that adjustment may include a temporary worsening of some symptoms.

Unless your skin has a violent, allergic reaction, it is a good idea to try new products for a full month. When you do change to a new product, only change one thing at a time.

If you change everything all at once, it will be hard to pinpoint which part of the change is working well and which may be causing problems.

As women age and hormone levels change, acne often flares up. Acne treatment in mature women may be different than acne treatment for teens.

While teens often use very drying products, this can be disastrous for a mature woman because it will cause excessive drying to skin that is not affected by acne. This could result in irritation and rashes that are just as unappealing as blemishes.

Look for products that are gently astringent and provide oil free hydration to the skin. Natural products include aloe Vera gel and honey.

Be sure to protect your skin and hair from the ravages of the sun. If you will be out in the sun for an extended period of time, be sure to use a good sunscreen and reapply it as directed.

Keep a sun hat and a light, long sleeved wrap on hand to shelter your hair, face, neck and arms from the sun if you find you are caught out unexpectedly.

Carrying a parasol is becoming more popular with the advent of global warming, and it is a good way to protect you from the sun and give yourself a cool spot of shade.

Further, consider your lifestyle habits in order to keep your skin looking its best. If you are a smoker, stop today.

Smoking damages even the deepest layers of your skin, and it makes you look sallow and sickly. Also make sure to manage your diet properly.

Eat foods that provide your skin with the vitamins and nutrients you need, and try to avoid processed foods that can add toxins to your body which will negatively influence the appearance of your skin.

Finally, do what you can to minimize stress in your life. Stress comes from many sources, and it can be healthy in small doses. With too much stress however, you will age your skin and feel unhealthy.

Stress can be reduced by spending time on yoga or meditation, taking some time to enjoy a warm bath nightly or practicing positive affirmations on a regular basis.

Even walking a pet or talking to a friend can help you to reduce stress levels. Whatever method you choose, make sure to address stress in a positive way to keep it from negatively influencing your appearance.

Your skin is a mirror to the inside of your body, and everything you do to yourself will influence its appearance.

Take the time to care for yourself properly in order to always look your best. This will go a long way toward keeping you young and beautiful for many years to come.

Your Home reflects your life

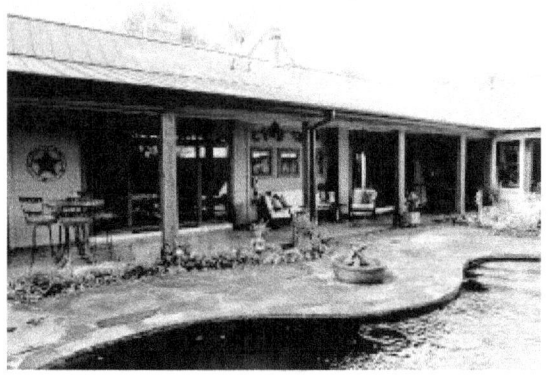

Every home tells a story. Your home will tell your story, things you take pleasure in, your feelings, attitudes, family, friends.

A home is a reflection of you, your experiences and knowledge. It expresses who you are, so create a home that is a reflection of how you want to live.

The little knick-knacks you have collected in your journey through life, find the perfect place in it.

The warmth and comfort you feel within is reflected in the way you arrange and display objects lovingly around your most-prized possession — your home!

If home reflects who you are; you are a mirror image of your home too. The condition of home psychologically influences your emotions, behavior patterns, attitude towards life and mental health.

Understand your vision

Look within for inspiration and motivation. Feelings that find meaning in your heart are manifested in the simple arrangement in your home; say the display of sunflowers near that sunlit window or the angle of your coffee table in the patio.

It is an extension of your moods, emotions and sentiments, what you hold most dear in that far corner of your heart.

Make wise choices

Different facets of your personality will go into creating a home that is a reflection of how you want to live. Once the key parts of yourself and your attitude have been identified, choices have to be made.

Decisions have to be taken, so choose wisely. The way you decorate (or choose not to), display pictures and objects, choose objects you want to be surrounded with, express what you are.

Create a home that is a reflection of how you want to live. Let your inner self shine through in your home. A healthy home doesn't have to be packed with designer furnishings created by hot decorators.

You want to live life in comfort and ease, so there should be a place for everything — a place to rest your tired legs, hang your bags and jackets, that favorite umbrella!

Those books you have collected over the years need a good display. They reflect the knowledge and experience you have gained over the years. The care that you put into your home expresses how you love yourself and life.

Reflections of emotions and dreams

Our home is exclusively our space. We may not realize it but it gives us ample opportunity for creative expression.

Just a shaft of sunlight, fresh air, bright colors and flowers will illustrate happiness. A cluttered house or closed curtains means sadness and a closed personality.

So you love your job? Reminders of work will be strewn around the house. Want a big vacation? Display pictures or objects that make your dreams come alive.

A visitor will interpret these symbols and signs as how you want to live. So be careful that they are real reflections of your hobbies, interests and habits.

Want to live life gardening? Have a green thumb? Be sure to have lots of plants and gardening tools around.

An escape, a showplace

Just close your eyes and think. How do you really want to live? Create a home that is a reflection of how you want to spend your life.

Is it where you want to escape the struggles of the big bad world, a warm place for family, showplace for possessions, entertainment? May be it is a mixture and balance is the key.

Find a place for every purpose — a place for family, public, your hobbies and displays. Do remember to designate a secluded space, a sanctuary where you unwind and meditate.

Smile through life

Every little thing, be it furniture or accessories, should be chosen with care. It should lighten up your face and bring happy thoughts of years gone by.

May be a gift with emotional value or that grandfather clock that has been in the family for generations? Be wary of keeping things that have no meaning for you. Just give them away.

Strike a balance

Steer clear of different styles. Choose one and stick to it. Strike a balance in color and style throughout the home. Place every article according to the functionality of the space and the activity for which it is to be used.

Scheming with colors

Understand the language of colors. Imagine the color wheel. The red side symbolizes passion, warmth, gaiety and even anger. It's not a good choice for the bedroom.

Yellow emanates positive energy and fills surroundings with warmth. The far side of the spectrum denotes coolness, reserve and is distant. Make a choice based on how you want to live.

Once you clearly understand the influence your environs exert, you can use the knowledge and experience to create a home that is a reflection of how you want to live. So go ahead and live life!

Be your own wellness CEO

At age 40, the risk of developing certain age- related diseases such as diabetes, stroke, and heart disease among others increase. However, the good news is that you can help keep the diseases at bay by following these health tips from medical experts.

Doctors recommend among others checking your family medical history and doing muscle-building exercises to prevent muscle loss. Below are ways you can maintain your health after 40

1. **Gauge yourself**

The first step in becoming your own wellness CEO is to know your numbers. Have your blood pressure, body weight, cholesterol levels and blood sugars checked.

Visiting your doctor to have these things checked will help identify potential problems early.

In addition, this is a good time to take a good look at your family history. Understanding your family history will help you know the diseases you need to look out for and take measures

2. **Improve your diet**

As we grow old, our metabolism slows down. You can improve your diet by:

· Reducing the number of calories you consume. Eating fewer calories will help boost your health. Since the metabolic rate is low, eating more calories than your body is able to burn will lead to accumulation of body fat.

· Eat more good fats- At age forty there is a tenderness of accumulating excess fats around the stomach.

Research shows that consuming foods high in monounsaturated fats such as nuts, avocados, and soybeans can help prevent the accumulation of abdominal fat.

Saturated fats and trans-fats found in baked and processed tend to lead to the accumulation of fats in the belly.

· Eat foods high in fiber- Incorporate more fruits, vegetables and whole grain foods. Eating foods such as pineapples, and oats with soluble fiber lowers the insulin levels, which speeds up the burning of fats.

· Drink enough water- Water is essential for helping get toxins out of the body. Drink at least eight glassed of water daily

3. **Exercise**

Starting age 40, people start losing about 1 percent of muscle per year. It's thus important to incorporate weight lifting exercises and cardio to help build muscle. Some of the best exercises to build muscle include

· Cardio exercises- Aerobic exercises such as running, swimming and biking can help improve flexibility, strength and overall balance.

· Resistance training- According to studies, combining cardio with resistance training is more effective to help build muscle mass and losing excess body fats.

It's advisable to talk to your doctor first for advice on the best workout for you and the ones you should avoid. Perform the above exercises three times a week.

4. Stress management

Too much stress often to stress related conditions including depression, obesity, among others. Learn to manage stress for a healthier life.

Some of the most effective approaches for stress management include getting enough sleep, meditation and avoiding stressors if you can.

5. Improve your lifestyle

Some lifestyle changes such as reducing alcohol and smoking or avoiding them altogether can go a long way in improving your wellness and life. Focus on eating healthy and avoid substances that can lower the quality of your life.

6. Train your brain

Studies show that performing brain-challenging games can help sharpen cognitive skills.

Stimulate your brain by playing chess, solving a puzzle or learning a new language. Keeping your brain active and learning new things can help prevent age- related memory loss

7. **Keep your social life alive**

Connect with family and friends. Socializing and spending time with loved ones can help reduce stress and help preserve your mental and physical health.

Studies show that social interactions keep the brain active, which helps prevent memory loss. In addition, humans are social beings and interaction is a basic human need. Remain active and participate in social activities

8. **Know what to watch out for**

Watch out for any health problems including pelvic pain, any tingling sensations, flu-like symptoms, shortness of breath among other symptoms. Learn to listen to your body and have any symptoms checked for diagnosis

As we grow older, it's important to take care of ourselves for a longer healthier life.

Maintain a proper diet, work out regularly, manage stress, and interact with others to help reduce stress and improve your mental health.

Simple lifestyle changes can go a long way in helping you enjoy a longer healthier life.

Life after 40

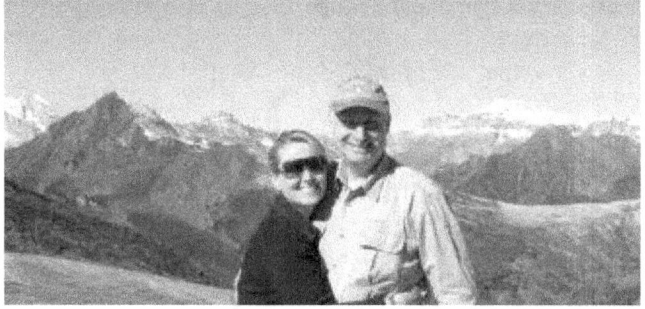

When most people stick their 40th candle on the birthday cake, it is more worrisome than joyful.

40 is the dreaded number when it comes to age because of quite a number of valid reasons. When you hit forty you have reached the apex of your life and so has the body.

From this point everything starts to sag and life starts to look slow. However, you should not let this factors wear you down. There are some ways you could buy yourself more time and make your life after 40 more productive.

Research suggests that every year after your 40th birthday, 1% of your muscle is turned to fat. This is a normal process of ageing. Because of this you eventually lose mobility if you grow older.

However, to slow down this process you can start exercising so as to make the muscles of your body relevant and stronger. Also, your body systems will slow down and as a result, your metabolism also slumps.

 This means that the amounts of calories that are processed by your body for intake also decline. After forty you are more likely to start gaining weight.

Exercising frequently will help burn the extra calories and give you a leaner and stronger body.

Work outs like jogging and squats are ideal for this purpose. This will give you some much needed confidence to continue living your life as you were before.

Naturally life after is all about making sure you don't look like you are forty. It is about becoming more concerned about what you consume so that it reflects well on your body.

After 40, most of the kids have moved out and your life has slowed down. At this point you are able to sit down and for once in a long time realize how helping others took a toll on you and your body.

To reverse this, you need to take a look at what you eat. Primarily you want foods that are rich in anti-oxidants that will help rejuvenate your skin cells and help fight free radicals.

You also want foods that are rich in nutrients and vitamins and you need to stay as far away from fast foods as you can.

After forty some women start experiencing menopause and a variety of other health conditions.

The immunity of the body also starts being less efficient and this could spell trouble if you were to suffer from some serious illness.

To keep this from happening, you need to have regular medical check-ups and make sure your doctor is among your best friends so to say.

It will help any diseases that are likely to creep in after 40 like breast cancer to get noticed early enough.

If you are a smoker, this would be a good time to quit. The same goes for alcoholics and also those that love the couch so much. At this juncture all your body needs is some good nutrients and all that is healthy.

Smoking and taking alcohol only serves to overwork some of your organs that are already starting to wear out not to mention that it also puts you at risk of contracting illnesses like lung cancer and Cirrhosis.

Being able to quit earlier could also be better and less harmful to your body. It would also be a good time to stock up on some good vitamins and omega supplements to help boost your nutrition and reduce the process of bone wasting.

Most people will agree that after 40 you sit down and analyze how the vicious world has changed you overtime.

This is also a good time to reflect on some the old teachings from your parents as they are exactly what you need. To begin with, laugh more. Surround yourself with people who make you happy.

This way you reduce chances of being stressed. Also prepare to help others as you help yourself. There is no better feeling than making someone feels good about themselves.

Since the kids have left home and are all grown, you need to keep busy. It will not only keep your mind occupied but also give you some much needed exercise as nothing makes you age faster than sitting around.

How you feel about yourself at this point greatly reflects on how you look. Don't sob over how slim and fit you looked at your 20s they are in the past and nothing is as good as the present.

Embrace your physique and invest in stylish clothes and shoes that are appropriate for your age. If you look good you feel good.

Remember that even though things don't spell very nicely when you hit past forty, how well you age and how well you look are still within your control. It is not the time to get disconnected with the world.

The best thing here is to work out more often, eat healthier, share joy and offer help where you can and above all stay in touch with your family. They will give you the strength, urge and love to move on.

They can also teach you about face book and other new things they will keep your mind active and occupied. Staying connected with current things will also help you feel much younger not to mention you will also seem much younger operating an iPod.